The Sirtfood Diet

The Complete Beginner's Guide For Rapid Weight loss and a Healthy Life. Includes Delicious Recipes to Activate Your Skinny Gene and Everything You Need to Know About Sirtfood Diet

Emre D. Blake

Table of Contents

Chapter 10: Treat and Dessert Recipes

Healthy Brownie Bites
Chocolate Coconut Bites
Chocolate Mousse
Chocolate Coffee Bites

Conclusion

Introduction

Have you decided that it is time for you to lose weight? Maybe you have tried in the past but felt like you did not get anywhere. Perhaps you felt like the diets that you were trying were too restrictive, limiting, or otherwise something that you did not want to comply with. Maybe you felt like the diet was just not right for you because you did not like the foods that you were told to consume. No matter the reasoning, however, you may have given up in the past. You may have come to the conclusion that you are stuck with your weight, whether you want it or not.

You do not have to be uncomfortable in your own skin. You can learn how you can lose weight without cutting out foods that you enjoy. Do you like red wine? Do you like dark chocolate? These are often cut from diets, claiming that they are unhealthy or unproductive. They are oftentimes removed so that people can focus on healthier foods or on foods that are less calorie-dense. However, what fun is it if you have to give up things that you love? If a diet is meant to be a lifestyle, why would you want one that will block out some of the foods and drinks that you like the most?

Thankfully, with a wide range of diets that are available to you in the world, you have choices. You can choose whether you want to cut out all carbs or cut out all fat. You can choose whether you want to go on a keto diet—but let's be real: Why is it okay to eat bacon and drink vodka, but it is not okay to enjoy an apple or drink red wine? Red wine itself is often touted as being full of diet-friendly antioxidants that should be consumed, sometimes regularly, according to the Mediterranean Diet. Diets should not feel restrictive. They should not make you feel like you are missing out or that you are not getting what you want. They should make you feel good about yourself; otherwise, they are not going to stick.

All too often, diets fail when the individual on a diet feels like they cannot get what they want. They feel like they cannot enjoy what they actually care to, and then when they unintentionally slip up at some point along the way, they feel like they cannot get back on the bandwagon. That happens and leaves people feeling like they cannot stick to it. They feel like there is no point if they already fell through, and soon, they are right back to binge-eating. Why waste your time working with a diet that is not going to help you achieve what you want? Why waste your time with a diet that you are not going to follow through with? Instead, shift over to the Sirtfood diet.

The Sirtfood diet has been recently touted by celebrities singing its praises. Singer Adele claimed that, on the Sirtfood diet, she lost nearly 100 pounds through exercise, this diet, and the famous Green Juice that you will be learning about in later chapters. It is designed to make use of sirtfoods—foods that are said to unlock fat loss and help aid in the prevention of disease as well.

If you want to lose weight while still maintaining your health and still getting to enjoy foods like chocolate and red wine, then this is the diet for you. This diet will help you make use of sirtuins, the proteins within the body that are designed to regulate the functionality of the metabolism. Certain plant-based foods are able to increase the number of sirtuins in the body, and that is believed to offer the changes in metabolism that will unlock the key to losing weight. On the Sirtfood diet, you get to enjoy foods such as red wine, strawberries, soy, green tea, dark chocolate, and more. You get to actually feel good while eating real, good foods that will help you.

Through the alternations between restricting calories and eating sirtfoods, you are able to trigger the body to create more sirtuins, therefore unlocking your ability to lose weight quickly and easily. Even after you have gotten to the weight that you want, it is highly recommended that you continue to make use of these foods and green juice to help you stay healthy. The process of using sirtuins to lose weight ought to keep your muscle mass the same, and they also help you to provide yourself with a healthy body that you know will be better able to withstand getting ill.

Is it effective? You will have to decide yourself, but research suggests that it may truly be a way in which you can begin to rapidly lose weight to help you achieve that healthy body that you deserve. Within this book, you will be guided through coming to understand the Sirtfood Diet and how it works. You will see why it is so popular and the benefits that can come from consuming these sirtfoods. You will see how the Sirtfood Diet really works and what the best foods that are high in sirtuins are so that you can begin to plan your diet around them. You will talk about how you can get started on the Sirtfood diet, and finally, you will be provided with several recipes for breakfasts, lunches, dinners, snacks, and treats that you can enjoy when on the Sirtfood diet. We eat food to survive—but that does not mean that eating should not be enjoyable! When you consume these foods, you will find that ultimately, the Sirtfood Diet is one that you can begin to enjoy and see real benefits and results from.

Remember, before altering your diet in such a drastic way, it is important for you to consider your own current health. If you currently have eating restrictions, such as allergies, you may want to double-check that the foods that you will be eating are not going to trigger them. If your dietary restrictions are related to other issues, you may want to talk to your doctor prior to beginning so that you have a clear picture of your diet and whether this diet will be right for you. For the average healthy person with weight to lose, following these steps and adhering to this diet should not pose much of a problem, but if you are diabetic, pregnant or breastfeeding, or otherwise on food restrictions, you may want to evaluate to double-check that this diet will be right for you. Ultimately, your health is what will matter the most in this! You must make sure that you keep yourself healthy and strong!

Chapter 1: Defining the Sirtfood Diet

So, you are ready to lose weight, but you are not sure how. You are looking through diets online. You see the Mediterranean Diet. You see the Keto Diet. You see the Paleo Diet. There are countless options out there, all touting that they are the best because they will help you to lose weight quickly. Which one do you choose? You may scroll through them all without choosing one that seems right for you because you cannot think of one that is just right. You see all sorts of options, but none of them call out. Maybe you've tried Keto, but you missed your fruits and carbs too much. Perhaps you tried the Paleo diet, but it just was not doing it for you. Whether you have failed a diet in the past does not have to define the future for you; however—you can lose weight. You can learn how you can properly shed it off so that you will be able to love your own skin and stay healthier. Perhaps you just need a new way of making it work for you.

The Sirtfood Diet is a new diet that was designed in the UK, created by celebrity nutritionists, Aidan Goggins and Glen Matten, and published in a recipe book in 2016. Designed to allow for you to eat certain foods that will allow you to trigger your skinny gene, the diet is designed to help people rapidly shed the pounds without the same consequences that are commonly seen in other fad diets. Some diets require you to starve yourself and wind up, causing loss of muscle along with the fat. Others require you to give up on foods that you enjoy, making them so restrictive that they are difficult for most people to keep up with. However, the Sirtfood Diet encourages you to focus on sirtuin-rich foods that can be combined into meals that are delicious and satisfying. How does chicken curry sound? You can consume it on the Sirtfood Diet. What about a nice turmeric salmon? That is also a meal that you can enjoy. You can even enjoy blueberry pancakes for breakfast on this diet as well.

Within this chapter, we are going to take a look at the Sirtfood Diet. We are going to address what it is and whether it is effective. Finally, we will take a look at whether this diet is going to be right for you in the long run. This diet will involve phases of dieting, which will sometimes have you restricting calories down to 1000 per day, and that is not always safe for all people. However, if this diet is right for you, you will find that this could be a great option for you. Even if you cannot fully follow the diet, just enjoying these foods that are rich in sirtuins is a great way to support your diet and add all sorts of healthy foods to the mix.

What is the Sirtfood Diet

The Sirtfood Diet, as has been mentioned, is a diet in which you are able to provide yourself with higher than normal levels of sirtuin-rich foods so that you can use those sirtuins to activate the proteins within your body to teach it to be able to spur its own weight loss. When Goggins and Matten got together to study sirtfoods, they decided that they would experiment with them; they ultimately designed a diet that served to increase and maximize sirtfood intake while also encouraging mild calorie restrictions. Together, they found that on average, participants who took this challenge consumed the sirtuin-rich foods, and restricted their calories to between 1000-1500kCal per day were actually able to see impressive weight loss, even without any increase in exercising or activity. On average, during that first week, the members lost 7 pounds without doing much else other than changing their diet. Does that sound promising to you?

Even better, these people reported that they were able to gain muscle rather than losing it—something that is practically unheard of in the diet world. Typically, weight loss comes with muscle loss as well, but these individuals built it. They also reported that they were happier and healthier in general—their mental health and general wellbeing increased as well.

Overall, there are some pretty compelling reasons to start considering the Sirtfood Diet—if you want to lose weight, gain muscle, and be healthier, and this is a great way to be able to do this. It will take diligence and dedication, but if you can make sure that you commit to this process, you, too, can reap these benefits. You can begin to be a healthier individual, inside and out.

This diet will provide you with a general plan that you can follow—you have certain meals that are good for certain points in the cycle. Sometimes, you will want to restrict calories down to 1000 for a few days to allow your body to feel that mild to moderate restriction, and then you must increase to 1500 calories to ensure that you are providing your body with enough to give you energy and health. When you can do this, you will be facilitating those proper conditions that will create the effect t that you are looking for.

This diet is designed to take a three week period, at which point, you are encouraged to continue consuming the sirtfoods and drinking green juice. However, you repeat those first two phases again if you feel like doing so is the right choice for you as well. Whether you are vegetarian, vegan, or meat-loving, you can make this diet work for you. All you have to do is follow the guidelines that you will be provided with shortly.

Is the Sirtfood Diet Right for Me?

Now, you may be wondering if the Sirtfood Diet is right for you. It may be—if you are healthy otherwise and you know that you are able to tolerate those calorie restrictions, then this diet will probably be just fine for you. Do you have the dedication and the willpower to follow it? There is nothing worse for your weight-loss attempts than failing to see progress or failing to stick to it, so if you feel like you cannot make this diet work for you, you may not be in the right place.

Something to consider if you are interested in this diet is the fact that you will need a juicer—you need to be willing to go out and purchase one, which will often be somewhat pricy. Likewise, if you are on a limited budget, the pricier ingredients could pose a problem for you. It is important for you to consider that ultimately, the diet itself should be safe for most people, with the exceptions being those who already have dietary restrictions and people who are currently pregnant or breastfeeding. If you have a condition that requires you to *not* restrict calories, this would also not be for you. However, otherwise, you are likely to find that this diet will be perfectly fine for you in most situations, so long as you do feel comfortable with the restrictions.

Remember, even if you do not or cannot follow through with the restrictions, there is still a great benefit to adding the sirtuin-rich foods to your diet. As we will address shortly, many of the foods that you can get in that are rich in sirtuins are already highly nutritious and recognized as dietary powerhouses. There is no doubt about it—the foods that you will consume during this diet are good for you. They are very healthy and they should be included in your diet whether you want to follow the Sirtfood Diet or not.

Chapter 2: The Benefits of the Sirtfood Diet

While it is still fully researched and explored, the evidence currently points out that there is a wide range of benefits to the use of sirtuin activation. You can see all sorts of dietary benefits to this particular regimen that will overall make you a much healthier person. Currently, it is believed that you can find all sorts of real, compelling benefits if you made use of this diet on the regular, and that is promising. Let's go over some of the most common benefits now, and keep in mind that as of now, there is evidence to suggest this, but more research will need to be done over time.

You Will Lose Weight

The most obvious of the benefits is that you will lose weight on this diet. Whether you are exercising or not, there is no way that you would *not* lose weight when you follow the diet to a T. This diet will have you restrict your calories enough that anyone would lose weight. The average person uses around 2000 calories per day, and this diet will work to have you cut that in half; you will be providing yourself with just 1000 or 1500 calories based on the phase that you are in.

Weight loss is caused by a calorie deficit—it is as simple as that. When you restrict your calories, but you keep your metabolism up, you will find that you will naturally lose weight. This is normal. However, usually, that weight loss is a mix between fat and muscle. As you lose weight and muscle, you would then naturally see your metabolism slow as well. Of course, this means that over time, your weight loss plan is not nearly as effective as it was supposed to be, and as a direct result, you will have to cut calories further to keep that deficit between consumed calories and the calories that your body naturally burns. This means that weight loss eventually slows, or even plateaus if all you do is make use of a weight-loss regimen through cutting calories. You will lose muscle if you are not careful with the weight loss regimen and that will work against you.

However, thanks to the fact that you do not lose muscle mass during the Sirtfood Diet, you do not have to worry about this problem; you simply continue to lose weight because you are able to maintain your metabolism at levels that will be conducive to you continuing to lose that weight.

Your Appetite Will Slow

Though your first few days you may find that you are ravenous as your body adjusts to its new normal, over time, you should find that your diet will begin to slow down. Your body will adjust to the restrictions in calories, and you will be okay with the lower calorie days, especially because the food that you will be eating will include nutrient-dense food that will help your body feel like it is more satisfied. Lentils and buckwheat are very dense foods that are featured heavily in this diet, and you are able to add healthy fats, such as olive oil, to your diet so that you can feel truly satisfied, knowing that ultimately, you have given yourself enough to keep your body going. You will find that you will be able to tolerate the lower amounts of food, and that is a huge plus.

You, Will, Build Muscle

The sirtuins that you will be consuming will help you to keep your muscle mass up, and that is highly beneficial. Most diets will see you losing muscle mass, but when you make use of these Sirtfoods, you will find that there is surprising staying power for your muscles. Not only will it help you to hold on to the muscle that you already have, but you will also be seeing an increase of muscle as well.

Studies have shown that sirtuins can help boost muscle mass, especially in elderly individuals. A study done on aging mice showed that the sirtuin rich diet helped allow for the development and growth of blood vessels and muscle. This would then boost the energy that the elderly mice had by upwards of 80%. That is *massive.* If you want to make sure that your metabolism stays regulated, you must make sure that your muscles are there to help you, and if they are not, you can run into all sorts of problems. This means that if you really want to find a diet that will help you gain muscle and burn fat, the sirtuin-rich Sirtfood Diet may be one of the best for you.

You Can Control Blood Sugar

Sirtuin-rich foods are known to inhibit the release of insulin in fasting states. This will essentially allow for the management of blood sugar. With the use of sirtuins, you are able to essentially prevent your blood sugar from dropping too low. This is a great point to keep in mind as compelling for completion of this diet, especially when you recognize that ultimately, you want to maintain that blood sugar so that you feel functional when restricting calories. When you restrict calorie consumption, you run into other problems, such as not being able to properly manage your blood sugar. Have you ever skipped a meal or two and felt dizzy or weak? That is the impact of lower blood sugar—but the sirtuins will help you to regulate that out so that you feel strong enough to proceed forward without more foods.

You Can Decrease the Risk in Chronic Disease

The antioxidants that are provided in most of the sirtfoods are great at defending your body from suffering the effects of cancer or other chronic diseases. They are incredibly beneficial for the body—they are designed to protect your body from free radicals that are created as harmful byproducts to breaking down food or being exposed to radiation. The antioxidants work to protect your cells against these sorts of cells that will harm you, and because they do that, they can help reduce your risk of heart disease, cancer, or other common diseases that are suffered today.

Essentially, antioxidants work because they protect the body; many plant-based foods are rich in antioxidants, and they are quite powerful. The body itself cannot properly remove those free radicals that you will be exposed to overtime. It is impossible not to be—even the sun will leave you being exposed to radiation every time that you leave your house. The free radicals and oxidative stress have been linked to problems such as Parkinson's disease, arthritis, and strokes. There are also many inflammatory conditions that are believed to be related to these free radicals.

It May Be Anti-Aging

Finally, studies are being done to explore whether this could have an anti-aging effect on the body, and so far, signs are showing that it may. Consider the increase in muscle volume; for example; the fact that it is something that people are able to latch onto is powerful and protective. The increase is something that you will find is able to help the body resist aging just by virtue of it being in effect. For example, think of many ailments of the aging population. Osteoporosis—the weakening of bones is one such example, and the increased muscle mass can help to fight off the bone fractures that would come with it. Likewise, the clearing of free radicals may also help to slow down the aging process as well—this is why so many diets push this anti-aging process.

Chapter 3: How the Sirtfood Diet Works

Now, this all may sound too good to be true at this point in time. How is it potentially possible that you can do all of that just with the use of the Sirtfood diet? How can you ever hope to change the way in which your body will respond to the calorie restrictions? If most of the time, fasting and calorie restriction impacts the metabolism, how is it that sirtfoods would not? These are all very important questions to keep in mind, and if you are looking at doing something to your body, such as restricting calories, you are absolutely in the right, asking questions about how what you are doing will work and impact your body. Rest assured—your questions will be answered. Here, we are going to answer four key questions. What are sirtuins? How do sirtuins work for the body? How does calorie restriction impact the body? What are the effects of eating sirtuin-rich foods? As you read, hopefully, you will get an idea of what it is that you can come to expect if you decide that this is the diet for you.

What are Sirtuins?

Sirtuins is the name for a whole host of proteins that are there to regulate the health of your cells. They help your body to maintain cellular homeostasis, which is a fancy way of saying that they keep the cells balanced to the specifications that they are supposed to be. Homeostasis is found when your body has functions that keep it in the same condition constantly, which is why your body is usually always at right around 98.6 degrees Fahrenheit—that is a way that your body maintains homeostasis. Likewise, your cells have a process to keep them in homeostasis as well—the sirtuins.

Proteins in your body are the workers, essentially, they work to serve very specific roles to keep your body functioning. Think of your body as one big corporation. Within your body, you have different sorts of parts; there are the organs, which serve sort of like the management of a corporation. You have nerves, which connect everything together like a network of computers. You have proteins—these are like individual departments within your particular corporation. Think about it—a corporation will have customer service, human resources, and all sorts of other departments within it so that it can function properly. They are all departments—but they are each responsible for a different role. Proteins in the body are similar; they are like the departments that keep everything going. When you take a look at sirtuins, you are looking at a department of proteins that is capable of providing your cells with a way that it can keep the body functioning. In terms of the Sirtfood Diet, they are recognized as the parts that can activate the "skinny gene"—they tell your body to let go of the fats.

How do Sirtuins Work?

You have seven sirtuins in your body—three of them are designed to work in the mitochondria, three of them work in the nucleus, where your DNA is stored so that cells can be run and regulated, and one more is kept in the cytoplasm. They all work together and have very different roles, but they all do one thing: remove acetyl groups from proteins.

Acetyl groups are able to alter and control the reactions that a cell has—they are like barcodes on proteins that tell other proteins what they are and how to interact with them. Through the process of deacetylation, sirtuins work to recognize that a molecule in the body has an acetyl group and they then move it, allowing the molecule to get ready to do its job. Essentially, the sirtuins are able to get everything ready to work.

In terms of the Sirtfood Diet, then you can expect that the act of fasting and restricting calories will change the way that the body is working. It will then allow for the sirtuins throughout the body to have an effect on how it works. Fat synthesis is repressed. The body is told not to uptake the cholesterol. The body is able to reject the fatty acids. Because fasting will up the level of activation of sirtuins, it allows for fats to not be stored. They are activated for use instead, allowing the body to burn them for energy when it is needed. The barcodes for those acetyl groups on the fats in the body essentially get scanned, and the sirtuins tell the molecule to get ready for work—which in this case, will be making use of the way that the body processes it. The fat goes through oxidation, gets used up, and therefore is lost from the body.

What Happens When I Restrict Calories?

When you restrict calories, you essentially tell your body that food is not available to it. You have a normal metabolism that is meant to tell you when to eat to make sure that you constantly have energy. Think of hunger like that little gas light coming on in your car—it is there to remind you that you are running low on stored gas and that filling it up soon would probably be a good idea. Your hunger is there to essentially keep you topped off—it does not want you to drop below a certain level. However, when you restrict your calories, you do not provide that extra food. This means that your body has to shift gears—it can no longer count on being topped off to provide the energy levels that are needed, and the deficit is created.

When that happens, the body has a great back-up mechanism that your car does not. Your body has stores of fat that can be broken down when there is a deficit in calories. When your body cannot get what it requires, it is able to instead work to get those calories elsewhere; it is able to provide itself with energy by breaking down that fat. Does that sound familiar? It is quite like the function of the sirtuins! Essentially, due to the threat to homeostasis in the body, the sirtuins activate and inhibit insulin while encouraging the oxidation of the fat in the body.

Usually, during calorie restriction, there are also other side effects, such as losing muscle, but that will be able to be protected against in other ways. During mild to moderate calorie restriction, weight loss is normal and expected without too many other issues. One of the more common ways of creating a deficit in calories is through the use of exercising while also restricting calories.

What Happens When I Eat Sirtuin-Rich Food?

When you eat sirtuin-rich foods, you are bringing more of those sirtuins into your body and therefore have more access to them for breaking down and using. This is highly beneficial to you—you will have them readily available in your body to be able to use them. Even more beneficial, however, is the fact that so many of the foods that *are* rich in sirtuin are typically also highly healthy for you. As you will see in the next chapter, you are looking to consume primarily all sorts of fruits and vegetables that will help you to keep your body happy, healthy, and ready to tackle the world.

Sirtuin rich foods are typically foods dubbed "superfoods"—those that are full of all sorts of what your body needs to survive and thrive. The increased nutrient content in these foods on their own is already a compelling reason to add them into your diet—the addition of the sirtuins is just icing on top. Remember, the Sirtfood Diet is all about healthy eating—it is meant to keep your body healthy with the rapid weight loss being secondary to it.

Chapter 4: Common Foods Found in the Sirtfood Diet

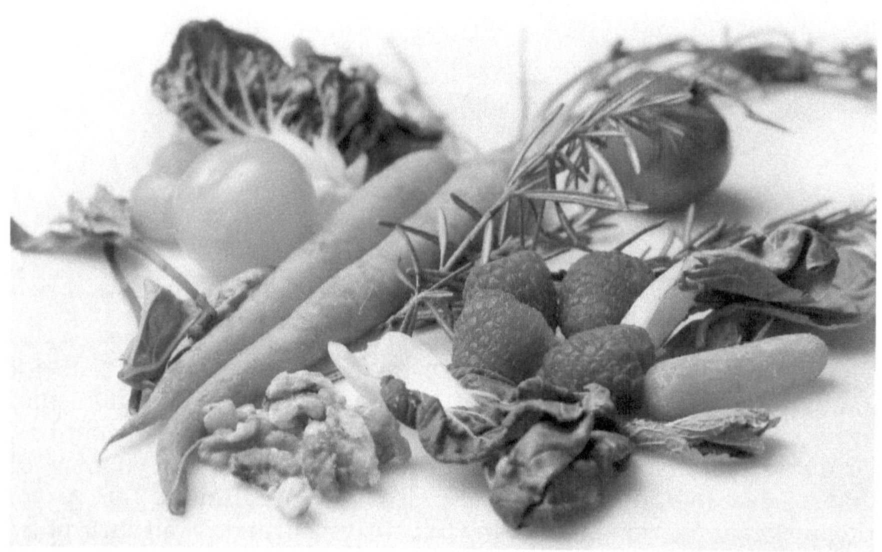

Now, you may be wondering so far what it is that makes up the Sirtfood Diet. What foods can you look forward to consuming when you make use of this diet? What is so compelling about them that makes people stick to it? Thankfully, as you read through this list, you will probably find that a lot of these are already pretty easy for you to include in your diet. They are common enough foods or staples, and you never even realized it. If these foods are already in your diet, you should pat yourself on the back—and then add more of them. These foods will be your bread and butter during the time that you are going to be maintaining your diet. Thankfully, you have red wine, chocolate, and coffee, three of the more common no-no's in other diets as being completely acceptable within this diet.

The ingredients that you will use in the later chapters to make use of this diet are going to be drawing heavily from this list. This is because they are quite healthy and if you want to, you can simply implement the diet just by boosting up these foods. While the Phase 1 and Phase 2 stages will absolutely help with weight loss, if all you want to do is eat healthier and get the benefits of the sirtfoods, then simply adding the ingredients to your diet is probably going to help you far more than you realize.

Now, let's go through and meet the ingredients that you will get to know over the next several weeks. We will go over the ingredient, why it is good for you, and common usage of it in general meals.

Red Wine

Not everyone is willing to consider alcohol as something that is healthy, but in moderation, it is believed that red wine is something that can be good for you. Alcohol itself may not always be the best choice, but it is believed that alcohol is something that is protective against problems with the blood vessels in your body. Further, red wine is filled up with antioxidants that will help your body to stay nice and healthy over time. In particular, wine has resveratrol—an antioxidant that is believed to lower the levels of LDL ("bad" cholesterol) in your blood while also reducing inflammation and preventing blood clots. Consuming in moderation, such as few drinks per week, will likely do more good than harm.

Dark Chocolate

Dark chocolate, like wine, is filled up with antioxidants. In fact, it is one of the best sources that you can get if you want to load up on those antioxidants—you can get a wide range of health benefits by switching from milk chocolate to dark chocolate. At higher levels (85% is recommended for the Sirtfood Diet), this is actually incredibly healthy for you. A 100-gram bar, which is admittedly on the larger side for a serving, clocking in at 600 calories worth of chocolate, can provide you with 2/3 of your iron intake for the day. It will also provide almost 60% of your magnesium, almost 90% of your copper, and almost 100% of your manganese, while also being high in potassium, zinc, phosphorus, and selenium. Likewise, it gets all sorts of benefits from its antioxidant content, and you can expect to see a wide range of health benefits. Of course, due to the sugar, you would probably want to consume in moderation.

Strawberries

Strawberries are another great source of sirtuins that also provide you with a wide range of benefits. Whether you eat them straight without preparing them, include them in a salad, toss them in yogurt, or have any other preferences to how you wish to consume them, there is no doubt about it—strawberries are beneficial. All you have to do is consume them. Strawberries are also high in antioxidants that are great for your heart and blood sugar. They are also quite rich in vitamin C, folate, and manganese. They are deemed a superfood for a reason and they will leave you feeling better than ever.

Kale

Kale is perhaps one of the greatest, healthiest veggies that you can take advantage of—for good reason. It is by far one of the healthiest foods that you can get, and it happens to also be a wonderful source of sirtuins. It may be a bit of an acquired taste, but over time, you can grow to love it—and you will also probably find that it is highly beneficial to your health as well. Eaten on its own, sautéed, as chips, or mixed into a salad, kale is something that you should try to consume regularly. Even better, kale is low in calories while also providing a massive amount of your nutritional value, meaning that you get the best bang for your buck, especially when you are busy restricting calories. One cup of kale, roughly 33 calories, will have over 200% of your daily value of vitamin A, nearly 700% of your vitamin K, 130% of vitamin C, and is loaded up with all sorts of other essentials as well. It also happens to be loaded up with antioxidants like beta-carotene, helping to clear out the body and offering very similar benefits to those that you can expect to see in the Sirtfood Diet.

Arugula

Arugula is part of the same family that also houses kale and is also sometimes referred to as rocket. It provides high levels of antioxidants within it as well, and it has been found that the higher levels of nitrate within them can also aid in blood pressure and the need for oxygen in exercise. In fact, it can actually even help athletes and their performance. Like kale, it can be expected to be used cooked or in salads, or also as a garnish on sandwiches. It is tender and tangy, and that makes it a great option for many people who want something a little less bitter than kale.

Onions

Onions may be stinky and they may make you cry, but they are fantastic sources of vitamins and minerals that cannot be forgotten about. When it comes right down to it, they are highly nutrient-dense and loaded up with all sorts of those very same antioxidants that you have seen throughout this chapter so far. Even better, the addition of onions to tomatoes is believed to aid the boost that you get from the lycopene in tomatoes, another source of antioxidants to boost that effect as well. Thankfully, tomatoes are delicious and made even better together with sandwiches, in sauces, on pizza, and more.

Matcha

Matcha is also rich in antioxidants—this time in catechins. This particular tea is able to help protect the liver and boost the power of the brain. It is able to help boost your metabolism, energy, levels, and protects against cancer. It has been found that this, too, lowers the levels of LDL cholesterol, and it can also aid in the detoxing of the body, allowing for many of those negative, unhealthy chemicals to be released. This is also a natural weight loss booster, thanks to the way that it does work to help promote weight loss. This is particularly prevalent in the green juice that you will be learning about soon and will be a major factor in your diet that you will want to keep on hand constantly.

Parsley

Most people do not think of parsley as particularly healthy or even think of it at all when it comes to food just due to the fact that it is not really needed to be consumed on its own. Rather, it is used typically in small amounts as a garnish on food. However, many people are then missing out on all of the wonderful health benefits that parsley has to offer. It is high in vitamins A, C, and K, and it is also once again, high in antioxidants. You will see this added into the green juice as well.

Soy

Soy may be somewhat controversial, but it is highly healthy as well, and it will serve as a wonderful plant-based protein for your meals as you read through the recipes that will be provided to you. You will be able to introduce the plant protein to your diet, meaning that you are getting food that is lower in fats and loaded up with omega-3 and omega-6 fats, which you will need.

Blueberries

Blueberries, fresh, frozen, cooked, or otherwise incorporated, are also full of all sorts of vitamins and minerals that you will need. They are good for your heart, your bones, your skin, and more. They can aid in the regulation of blood pressure and sugar, and they can even be good for your mental health. Overall, blueberries are a wonderful option to add into your diet, but be mindful as the vitamin K content can interfere with blood thinners. This fruit is also loaded up with antioxidants that help them be the healthy powerhouse that they are. If you are craving something sweet, this is a great way to get that added to your diet, and they can be added into your oatmeal or pancakes as well to get some extra taste.

Lovage

Lovage is a little-known leafy plant that is quite similar to parsley—it is a small, fragrant herb that can be used medicinally regularly. It is used to help with inflammation typically, as well as serves as a diuretic. This is one of the ingredients that you will be encouraged to throw into your juice. Beware that it is potentially unsafe if used during pregnancy—especially in the early stages, it has been found that it may be linked to contractions of the uterus, which could also cause miscarriage. Thankfully, this is an optional addition to your green juice, and you are free to skip it if you choose to do so.

Coffee

Coffee is popular for a reason—the caffeine is a wonderful natural boost to energy ad; there is also a whole slew of health benefits as well. In particular, you can find that you will be able to prevent diseases through the use of coffee. It is full of all sorts of antioxidants that can help release the occurrence of all sorts of health concerns, such as heart disease. It is also found to be used as a natural fat burner—it can help you boost your metabolism up to 10%. It is also full of vitamins B2, B5, potassium, manganese, and magnesium. Moderate caffeine usage is fair game in this diet, and even better, coffee, when plain, is virtually calorie-free. While some diets may recommend avoiding caffeine or coffee, it is deemed one of the major sirtfoods to consume in this particular diet, meaning that you are free to consume them as much as you would like.

Capers

Capers are commonly used in food as a side to proteins and are a delicious way to add some variety to your diet. However, they also help through the use of adding antioxidants to your diet, much like how the rest of the ingredients so far have

benefitted you. If you want to be able to thrive on this diet, these are a great way
to add some extra flavor. They are slightly acidic and delicious. You can expect
these to be found in jars in the pickled area in your grocery store, and if you do
decide to buy them, you can add them to salads or in other meals as a side.

Turmeric

Turmeric pops up repeatedly in all sorts of diets and for a good reason—it is
incredibly beneficial to all sorts of people for all sorts of reasons. If you want to
add a natural nutritional supplement to your life, this is it. It is highly beneficial
to your brain and your body, and even better, it tastes great. Turmeric is full of
curcuminoids, antioxidants that can be used to help you keep your body healthy.
Turmeric is filled up with this. However, it also aids in inflammation and,
therefore, would be able to help with many of the chronic diseases suffered from
in the western world. Even better, it boosts the ability of these powers to work by
blocking free radicals and then boosting your own antioxidant enzymes to help
fight against them. Essentially it is like the backup to the rest of the ingredients
while also providing high levels of antioxidants. Even better, you can throw it
together to make delicious curry with many of the other ingredients on this list so
far.

Walnuts

Walnuts are, you guessed it—rich in antioxidants. Even better, however, they also
have the addition of omega-3 fatty acids and can help you stay fuller for longer.
Whether you will eat handfuls on their own or mix them into anything else, this is
a great way for you to help support your body in staying happy and healthy. Most
often, these foods are eaten plain, but you can make use of them in all sorts of
other contexts, such as in your pasta or cereal, or baking them into something.
However, because they are high in fat, you will have to worry about the calorie
content if you are eating them during calorie restriction. Be mindful of how many
you are eating to ensure that you do not go over them when you are eating.

Extra Virgin Olive Oil

If you have to get oil for cooking, extra virgin olive oil (EVOO) is the one for you.
It is incredibly heart-healthy and also provides you with all sorts of other
vitamins and minerals that you will be able to make use of if you consume it. It is
naturally anti-inflammatory and also provides protection from heart disease and
inflammatory diseases. It is also found that olive oil itself is not linked to an
increase in weight—in fact, it can actually be tied to weight loss instead. You can
cook with it or toss some on top of some tomatoes or eat it any other way—it is
healthy for you no matter what you do to it. Again, remember moderation is key
because it is high in calories as it is still an oil.

Buckwheat

Buckwheat is a series of seeds, much like grains that are commonly used and
consumed as a replacement for other grains. You can use it and cook it like rice,
or you can eat it plain if you want. It is up to you. You will see this featured

heavily in this diet. However, it can be somewhat difficult to find on your own in the store, and you may have to order it online. This particular food is high in benefits as well—it is great at providing you with protein and fiber while also increasing energy and providing you with a reduction in blood pressure. You can also expect this particular food to help with weight loss as well, while also being highly satisfying to consume.

Chapter 5: Getting Started on the Sirtfood Diet

When you're ready to get started on the Sirtfood Diet, there are a few considerations that you need to keep in mind. You must understand what the phases are, what the maintenance will look like after completing the whole process, and what the green juice recipe is. The green juice is essential; you cannot complete the proper Sirtfood Diet if you choose to forego the juice, and because of that, you must make sure that you are able to get a high-quality juicer. You can find these usually for around $100 online or at any major department store.

Within this chapter, we are going to go over what you can expect, what you should be doing, and how to get through each of these stages. Then, we will talk about the maintenance that goes into what you do after you have finished losing the weight and you are satisfied with where you have ended up. These are important points to know so that you are able to provide yourself with everything that you will need to thrive on this diet. Remember, if you have any health concerns while on this diet, you should always consult a doctor.

Phase One

The first phase is the one that intimidates many people. During this phase, you are to cut your calories down from whatever you have been eating in the past to just 1000 calories per day. This is a hard limit; you must do this if you hope to be successful. This particular phase lasts seven days, during which you change your diet while still trying to maintain your usual daily schedule. This means that you should still work out if you were doing it before—you should still be walking and moving around to keep your body healthy, if at all possible.

The first three days of phase one require you to drink three green juices per day, followed by one sirtfood-heavy meal each day. You are to restrict your calories to just 1000 during this time. Remember, you are trying to activate those sirtuins in your body, and you need to make sure that you have a calorie deficit to make that happen.

During the last four days of this phase, you are to drink two green juices per day while eating two meals at 1500 calories per day. The meals must be rich in sirtuins, and still, you want to maintain the activity and the exercise as well as the calorie deficit. This is the time during which you are continuing to get your body ready to lose weight rapidly.

Phase Two

Phase two happens during the next two weeks. During this time, you are on a "maintenance" plan, but that maintenance plan is more along the lines of maintaining that deficit and the sirtuin activation that you saw in the other activations. When you use this particular stage, you are looking to continue to maintain that calorie deficit in hopes of being able to continue triggering your body to lose weight. You will be able to choose out your meals throughout this book, being mindful of what you choose, and how much of it you eat. If you do take into consideration what you are eating and keep active, you should find that you continue to lose weight.

After Finishing the Sirtfood Diet

When you have completed that three-week cycle, you have a few options for you—you can go back to phase one and complete it again if you are not comfortable with your weight yet. This is an option that you can do as much as you want until you *do* finish losing the weight that you are trying to shed. You will continue to work to shed the weight over and over again in hopes of getting rid of it.

Alternatively, you can choose to focus on simply eating foods rich in sirtuins without following the 1000 or 1500 calorie limits as well, while also working out. Remember, at some point, you will reach a weight that you want to maintain rather than continuing to facilitate weight loss, and when you get there, the best thing that you can do is to continue eating sirtuin-rich foods so that you know that you are getting everything that you need.

Whether you decide to continue to loop through the diet or you choose to stop losing the weight and instead focus on how you can maintain it, you will find that you can succeed with losing weight easily and making sure that the weight stays off. Remember, even just maintaining that healthy diet will be enough to help you to keep the weight off—all you have to do is remember to continue working toward it. Keeping a healthy weight is as simple as making sure that the calories balance out, and that is quite simple when it comes to using the sirtfood diet—one that is rich in healthy foods.

<u>Green Juice</u>

On this diet, you will have to get used to making and consuming green juice, which some people find to be delicious while others decide that they hate it. No matter, however, this is an important part of the diet. Keep in mind that the green juice contains matcha—a green tea powder that contains caffeine in it, so you will not want to add matcha if it is getting to be late in the day or you will not be able to sleep. You will drink this juice regularly and preferably daily, even after you have completed the diet; it is full of all sorts of good vitamins and minerals that will keep you healthy.

To make your green juice, you will first juice the greens, then add in the lemon juice by hand, and then you will add matcha and stir it into the juice. You can also fill it up to dilute it with water if you prefer to do so. Thankfully the recipe is quite simple.

Ingredients:

- 2 handfuls of kale
- 1 handful of arugula
- A small handful of parsley (preferably flat-leaf)
- (optional) a small handful of lovage
- 2 large celery stalks, leaves still attached
- ½ of a green apple
- Juice of half of a lemon
- A spoonful of matcha powder

To complete this recipe, you will need to do the following:

1. First, mix the greens together and add them to your juicer.
2. Then, rejoice, if necessary—leafy greens sometimes do not have the best results in juicers.
3. Then, juice the apple and celery.
4. Squeeze half of a lemon to remove the juice as well.
5. Mix well in your cup. At this point, you should have ~250 ml of juice.
6. Then, add matcha and dissolve.

Chapter 6: Breakfast Recipes

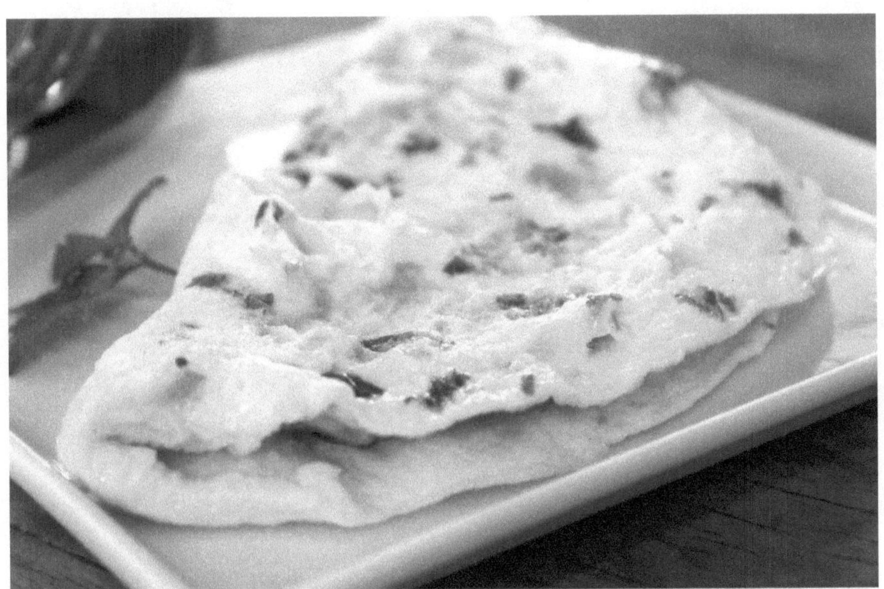

Mushroom Scramble

This is a great go-to breakfast if you want to eat a hearty, filling breakfast that is going to keep you going all morning. Even better, it tastes great and is simple to throw together—it will only take around 10 minutes to throw everything together and cook it. This recipe is enough to feed two people—if you are cooking for only yourself, cut it in half.

Ingredients:

- 4 eggs
- 2 tsp turmeric (ground)
- 3 tsp curry powder
- 2/3 cup chopped kale
- 2 tsp olive oil (extra virgin)
- 1 bird's eye chili, sliced (remove seeds if you prefer less burn)
- Button mushrooms sliced up—just a handful or two
- 1/3 cup of parsley, chopped

To complete this recipe, you will need to do the following:

1. Combine the turmeric and curry powder in a small bowl. Add a small amount of water and mix until it creates a paste
2. In a pot, steam your kale for just a few minutes—no more than 3

3. Heat the oil up on medium in a frying pan. Then, sauté the mushroom
   slices and the pepper slices. Wait for the mushrooms to start to soften.
4. Then, crack the eggs into the pan and mix with the spice paste. Cook the
   whole thing over medium heat for a minute and then mix in the kale.
5. Cook for another minute or until eggs are fully cooked. Then add the
   parsley to the pan, mix together to combine, and serve.

Date and Walnut Porridge

This is a simple, five-ingredient recipe that you can use to throw together to create a delicious porridge to get you started on the right foot. If you want a healthy meal for breakfast, this one can help greatly. This recipe is designed for two people. Cut it in half if you are only preparing for yourself.

Ingredients:

- 2 Medjool dates
- 100 g strawberries, washed, hulled, and chopped
- 8 chopped cup walnut halves
- 70 g buckwheat flakes
- 400 mL of milk of any kind (cow, goat, soy, almond, coconut, etc.)

To complete this recipe, you will need to do the following:

1. Add the milk into a pot with the dates.
2. Slowly heat it and then add in the buckwheat.
3. Continue to cook until the porridge is the right consistency for you.
4. Add in the walnuts and top with strawberries. Serve immediately.

Blueberry Banana Pancakes

Are you missing traditional breakfasts? Good news—you can make blueberry banana pancakes that are delicious and quite possibly, even better than traditional ones. All you have to do is substitute out a few ingredients for those that are healthier for you, and you will find that you have a delicious breakfast that you can probably even get your children to eat without complaint. This recipe is enough for you to serve 2-3 people; if you want more, then double the recipe.

Ingredients:

- 3 bananas
- 3 eggs
- 75 g rolled oats
- A pinch of salt
- 1 tsp baking powder
- ¾ cup of blueberries (fresh or frozen)

To complete this recipe, you will need to do the following:

1. Put your oats into a blender or food processor and pulse until you have created an oat flour.
2. Into your blender or food processor, add in everything but the blueberries. Pulse it together for roughly 2 minutes until it is well combined and you have a nice, smooth batter.
3. Pour the batter into a large mixing bowl and gently add in the blueberries, folding them in rather than mixing it up. Make sure that you do not overmix.
4. Wait 10 minutes, allowing the baking powder to activate.
5. Heat a frying pan to medium-high and add a small amount of oil or butter to the surface so that the pancake does not stick. Scoop in the blueberry banana batter to the size desired and allow it to fry until the bottom is golden brown and ready to flip.
6. Flip and cook the other side until also golden brown.

**Smoked Salmon Omelet**

This omelet is packed with delicious and healthy ingredients and packs quite the protein punch to keep you going throughout your day without worrying about missing out on those sirtfoods that you need. Featuring capers, arugula, parsley, and olive oil, this recipe is a great way to add those superfoods to your diet first thing in the morning. This recipe makes one large omelet for two people.

Ingredients:

- 4 medium eggs
- 1 1/3 cups sliced smoked salmon
- 1 tsp capers
- 1 ¼ cups chopped arugula
- 2 tsp chopped parsley
- 1 tsp olive oil for cooking

To complete this recipe, you will need to do the following:

1. Crack up the eggs into a bowl and combine. You must whisk well until well mixed.
2. Add all ingredients to the egg and mix well to combine.
3. Heat your olive oil in a frying pan until hot and shimmering, but not smoking on medium-high heat
4. Add the mixture to the pan and use your spatula to spread it evenly throughout
5. Reduce the heat to medium and wait for the omelet to complete cooking
6. When finished, use your spatula to roll or fold the omelet. Remove from heat, cut in half, and serve; ½ serves one person.

Veggie Omelet

Another option for you if you want to forego the fish is to create an egg and veggie mixture. This particular one will make use of veggies such as onion, bird's eye chili, and some arugula and kale, chopped up for you so that you can create a healthy breakfast to keep you satisfied throughout your day.

Ingredients:

- 4 eggs
- 2 tbsp olive oil to cook
- 1 small onion, chopped
- 1 bird's eye chili, diced
- A small handful of kale, chopped
- A small handful of arugula, chopped

To complete this recipe, you will need to prepare your ingredients. Then, complete the following:

1. Heat olive oil in a frying pan at medium-high heat
2. Cook the onions with the pepper until fragrant and the onions begin to turn translucent. Then, add in the chopped greens. Wait for them to wilt. Then, remove from the pan into a small bowl.
3. Crack eggs into a separate bowl and beat until mixed and combined. Salt and pepper to taste and then add the eggs to the frying pan, careful to spread them evenly.
4. After a minute of cooking, as the bottom of the egg starts to firm up, add the veggie mixture to the pan and spread them out on one half of the omelet. Then, fold the egg over the veggies. Slide onto a plate, cut in half, and serve.
5. Each half of the omelet serves 1 person.

Buckwheat Toasted Muesli

This recipe will create a toasted muesli with all sorts of wonderful, healthy nuts and grains that will keep you feeling full. You can use this for a wonderful addition to yogurt or porridge, or you could even add it to a smoothie or eat it plain. It is a delicious addition to nearly any diet and a wonderful option to have on hand. This will create a lot of muesli for you to use whenever you want. Add a few tablespoons to your food for a healthy, pleasant crunch.

Ingredients:

- 4 cups of puffed buckwheat
- 2 cups of buckwheat flakes
- 3 cups of walnuts, chopped
- ½ cup of melted coconut oil
- 1/3 cup of honey
- 2 tbsp cinnamon (ground)
- 2 tbsp vanilla extract
- 1 tsp salt

To complete this recipe, you will need to do the following:

1. Turn on the oven to 300 degrees Fahrenheit and preheat.
2. Combine your dry ingredients together and mix well.
3. In a pan, melt your coconut oil with your honey and vanilla. Wait for it to warm up to be runny, but do not let it boil or burn. It should just be runny.
4. Pour the liquid into the dry mixture and mix well until all ingredients are thoroughly coated
5. Spread out across the entire baking tray (lined with parchment paper)
6. Bake for 25 minutes, turning every 10 minutes to prevent burning
7. Remove from the oven and let it cool. It may not seem done at first, but be aware that it will crisp up when it is cool
8. When cool, move it to an airtight container. It should keep for about a month.

Strawberry Chocolate Chip Buckwheat Pancakes

Pancakes are a great option for breakfasts, and what do kids like in their pancakes more than chocolate chips? Well, there is an option for you to have that in your pancakes, too—dark chocolate that is. This is a great recipe that is healthy and Sirtfood Diet approved to start your breakfast with a bit of sweetness.

Ingredients:

- 1 cup of buckwheat flour
- 2 tbsp coconut sugar or honey
- 1 tsp baking powder
- 1 tsp cinnamon powder
- ¼ tsp salt
- ¾ cup of soy milk
- 2 tbsp olive oil (for cooking)
- 1 egg
- ½ cup finely chopped strawberries
- ¼ cup 85% dark chocolate, chopped finely (chips work as well)
- Any toppings you want

To complete this recipe, you will need to do the following:

1. Grease your skillet lightly and preheat it at medium heat
2. Mix your dry ingredients together, holding the chocolate chips and strawberries for later
3. Mix your wet ingredients together in a separate bowl, still holding the chocolate chips and strawberries
4. Mix in the strawberries and chocolate chips gently, folding them. Do not overmix
5. Using ½ cup of batter per pancake, add your first scoop to the skillet—you should get one that is roughly 5 inches wide
6. Cook for 5 minutes, or until the edges are cooking and it is bubbling on top. Flip, then cook another 2 minutes.
7. Repeat, lightly greasing your pan between pancakes—you should have four pancakes.

Overnight Buckwheat Porridge

This is a great overnight recipe that you can use to keep yourself full. While it does not contain any sugar itself, you can add the sweeteners yourself if you want some honey or agave within it—just try to keep the sugar low. This recipe is also vegan and can be topped with fresh fruit for a delicious addition.

Ingredients:

- 1 cup of buckwheat groats
- ¼ cup of chia seeds
- 3 cups of soy milk (you can sub this for any of the milk that you choose, cow's or otherwise)
- 1 cup of water
- A pinch of cinnamon
- A pinch of salt
- 2 tsp vanilla
- ½ cup crushed unsalted walnuts
- 1.5 cup chopped strawberries and blueberries

This recipe is incredibly simple to start the night before—all you have to do is the following:

1. Mix everything but the berries and nuts into a bowl, seal it, and leave in the fridge overnight.
2. When you are ready to eat it, pull it out, add it to a pot, and stir for 10-12 minutes over medium heat until it is the desired texture.
3. Add the fruits and nuts and serve.

Bacon and Arugula Omelet

Yes, another omelet is being added to your dish—this is a great one to eat if you are looking for something a bit heartier—the bacon can add some nice salt to the dish, and when you pair it with superfoods such as arugula, or even kale or spinach, you have something that is hearty and delicious. This serves two people—either set some aside for later or share it with someone at the moment.

Ingredients:

- 4 oz. bacon (usually about two slices)
- 6 medium eggs
- 2 cups of kale or arugula (or both), chopped
- 4 tbsp chopped parsley
- 2 tsp turmeric powder
- 1 tsp olive oil to cook

To complete this recipe, you will need to do the following:

1. Start with frying your bacon over medium or medium-high heat. Wait for the bacon to get crispy, then remove from a pan and place to drain the fat.
2. Clean the pan with a paper towel and set aside.
3. Add eggs to a bowl and whisk thoroughly. Then, add your chopped greens, your parsley, and your turmeric. Chop up the bacon and mix them into the mixture as well.
4. Add oil to pan and heat until hot and shimmery, but not smoky.
5. Add the eggs to the pan and swirl it around with the spatula. Continually mix the cooked egg until the raw egg is flat and even. Reduce heat to medium-low and wait for the omelet to finish.
6. Fold in half, remove from pan, cut in half, and serve.

Green Egg Scramble

This is a wonderfully healthy breakfast that can really add a perk to your step—all you have to do is prepare it and enjoy it. Filled with hearty eggs and the protein that you will need to keep yourself going, along with plenty of kale and arugula to really add those sirtuins to your diet, this is delicious. If you want a nice sirtfood breakfast, this is a wonderful one for you to enjoy and thrive with.

Ingredients:

- 3 cups of kale and arugula, chopped and packed
- 4 eggs
- 1/8 cup of sliced green onions
- 2 tsp fresh tarragon (chopped)
- 1 tbsp sour cream
- 1 tbsp butter (unsalted)
- 1 tbsp olive oil

To prepare this dish, all you need to do is:

1. Add your oil to a skillet on medium-high heat and wait until shimmering. Then, add the arugula and kale and a pinch of salt. Cook and toss occasionally until wilted—4 minutes usually. Remove spinach and set aside.
2. Wipe out the skillet and return to burner
3. Add eggs, chives, tarragon, and a pinch of salt and pepper to a bowl and whisk until well combined and starting to bubble.
4. Melt butter into a skillet on medium-high heat and add egg mixture. Stir slowly with a spatula until eggs start to set (1 minute or so). Add in the greens and fold them into the eggs until softly set.
5. Remove from heat and add the sour cream, gently folding it in. Serve.

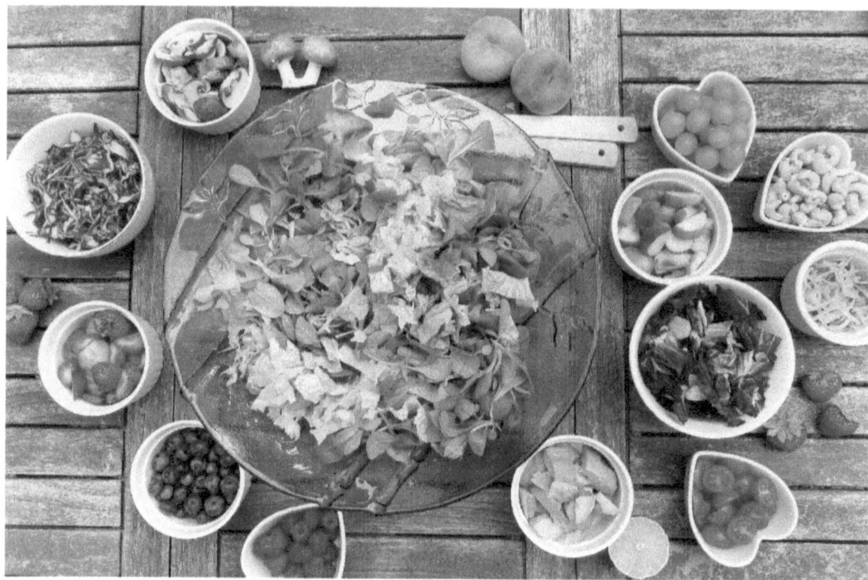

Lunchtime, especially during phase two and maintenance phase, can be a bit of a challenge if you do not have something that is easy to take with you to work each day. With many people working outside of the home most of the time, it is important that lunches are something that is easy and portable, and these recipes seek to do exactly that.

Green Juice Salad

Now, you may have gotten sick of the green juice, but let's be real—it is full of so many wonderfully healthy nutrients that can help you going and even better, all of those greens are full of fiber, meaning that when you eat this, you will get the bulkiness of the fiber to keep you feeling satisfied longer than with a liquid juice. Thankfully, this recipe is incredibly simple to throw together and you can take it with you to work if you want to in a Tupperware container for a quick, easy, healthy pick-me-up in the middle of the day.

Ingredients:

- 2 handfuls of chopped kale
- 1 handful of chopped arugula
- 1 tbsp chopped parsley
- 2 stalks of celery, sliced into bite-sized pieces
- ½ green apple, chopped into bite-sized pieces
- 6 walnuts, crushed
- 1 tbsp olive oil

- ½ lemon, juiced
- 1 tsp grated ginger
- A pinch of salt and pepper

To complete this recipe, you will need to do the following:

1. Mix the juice of the lemon, ginger, seasonings, and olive oil into a small jar or small Tupperware container. Set aside until you are ready to eat.
2. In a large bowl or large Tupperware container, add your kale, arugula, parsley, celery, apple, and walnut. Mix it up until well combined and set aside until you are ready to eat.
3. When you are ready to eat it, shake up your dressing, then add it to the bowl and mix thoroughly.

Strawberry Buckwheat Tabbouleh

This is a wonderful recipe that you can take and enjoy at work with ease and it comes straight from the Sirtfood Founders themselves as a suggestion. This salad only requires you to cook the buckwheat and then assemble the cooled salad and eat whenever works best for you. This is a double recipe—you can make two days for yourself or you can share it with someone else.

Ingredients:

- 2/3 cup buckwheat
- 2 tbsp turmeric powder
- 1 whole avocado, diced
- 1 whole tomato, diced
- ¼ cup diced red onion
- ¼ cup diced and pitted dates
- 2 tbsp capers
- 1 ½ cups roughly chopped parsley
- 1 1/3 cups sliced strawberries
- Juice from 1 lemon
- Two cups of chopped arugula

If you want to complete this recipe, you will need to do the following:

1. Cook your buckwheat with the turmeric powder added. Make sure that you follow the instructions that came on the package. When it is done, drain it and set it aside until it has completely cooled off
2. Mix all of your chopped ingredients together, keeping the arugula separate. Add the lemon and oil. Place all ingredients on top of the arugula and serve.

Salmon Salad

This next recipe is a delicious one, filled with all sorts of sirtfoods and bulked up with the presence of the salmon as well. Salads are a wonderful way for you to be able to bring your lunch with you on the go anywhere that you need to be and because of that, they can be great for you for workdays when you know that you will be hungry but will not have the space to cook right that moment. So long as you can keep this refrigerated, thanks to the salmon, you will be able to take this with you without it going off or bad or tasting funny.

Ingredients:

- 3 cups of arugula
- 3 cups of chicory leaves
- ½ cup sliced smoked salmon
- ½ of an avocado, peeled and sliced
- 6 walnuts, crushed,
- 1 tbsp capers
- 1 large Medjool date, pitted and chopped
- 1 tbsp of olive oil
- ¼ lemon, juiced
- 10 sprigs of parsley, chopped
- 1 medium stalk of celery, chopped
- ½ cup thinly sliced red onion

To complete this recipe, you will need to do the following:

1. Chop and prepare all ingredients
2. Place salad leaves into a large bowl
3. Mix the remaining ingredients together in another bowl and pour on top of the leaves. Serve.

Chicken Sirtfood Salad

If you are looking for a bit of diversity or maybe something with a bit more of a creamy tang to many of the other recipes, this is a great option for you. This recipe is there to provide you with chicken atop a bed of arugula to enjoy and as always, it is a great recipe to take with you on the go—all you have to do is mix it and prepare it. Make sure that this dish is kept refrigerated thanks to the dairy content if you are taking it with you to work.

Ingredients:

- ¼ cup plain Greek yogurt
- ¼ lemon, juiced
- 1 tsp cilantro, finely chopped
- 1 tsp turmeric powder
- ½ tsp curry powder (more to taste if you prefer it spicy)
- ¾ cup cooked chicken breast in bite-sized pieces
- 3 whole walnuts, crushed
- 1 Medjool date, pitted and diced
- 1/8 cup diced red onion
- 1 bird's eye chili, diced (remove seeds if you do not want it to be too spicy)
- 2.5 cups roughly chopped arugula

To make this recipe, you will need to do the following:

1. In a medium-sized bowl, combine your Greek yogurt, the juice from the lemon, your cilantro, and the curry and turmeric powders. Combine well.
2. Add in your chicken, walnuts, date, onion, and chili and mix together thoroughly.
3. Add to the top of the arugula. Serve.

Sirtfood Pesto Buckwheat Salad

This recipe is going to create a delicious Sirtfood-rich pesto that you can use atop your buckwheat pasta. If you want something that is a bit more substantial, you can make use of some chicken as well. Hot or cold, this pasta salad is a delicious meal on its own.

Ingredients:

- 4 cups of parsley
- 1 tsp minced garlic
- 1 lemon, juiced
- ½ cup of walnuts
- 3 bird's eye chilis—remove the seeds if you do not like spicy food
- ½ cup cauliflower, broken down
- 2 tbsp parmesan cheese, freshly shredded
- 2 tbsp extra virgin olive oil
- 2 tbsp water
- Salt and pepper to taste
- 2 cups diced chicken breast, cooked
- 8 oz buckwheat pasta (dry weight), cooked

To complete this recipe, you will need to do the following:

1. Prepare your chicken and pasta, and set aside in a large bowl.
2. In a food processor, combine all ingredients aside from chicken and pasta. Blend until the consistency of pesto. Stop and scrape down walls from time to time to mix well.
3. Add 1 cup of pesto to the pasta and mix. If still dry, add more pesto to taste and mix well. Store in the fridge until ready to eat. This serves 4.

Chicken and Kale Curry

Curry can be a great way to mix things up and try something with a different palate—and good news, curry is full of sirtuins, especially when you add kale or arugula to it. This recipe can be made ahead of time and stored in a tightly sealed container if you decide that you want or need to take it to lunch the next day. This recipe will produce curry for two servings.

Ingredients

- 1.5 cups boneless, skinless chicken thigh, raw and cut into bite-sized pieces
- ½ tbsp. olive oil
- 1 tbsp turmeric powder
- 1 whole diced red onion
- 2 cloves of garlic, crushed and minced
- 1 bird's eye chili, minced—remove seeds if you prefer something less spicy
- ½ tbsp. fresh ginger root, chopped
- ½ tbsp. curry powder (more to taste if you prefer it spicier)
- 1 cardamom pod
- 1/3 cup light coconut milk from a can (make sure it is the cooking kind, not the drinking milk substitute kind)
- ½ of a 14 oz can of chopped tomato
- ½ of a 14 oz can of chicken stock
- Cilantro for garnish

To complete this recipe, you will need to do the following:

1. In a glass bowl, add your chicken, 1 tsp of oil, and 1 tsp of turmeric. Combine, mix, and let it marinate. Use a spoon if you do not want stained fingers. Leave it in the fridge for at least 30 minutes.
2. Cook the chicken over medium heat in a frying pan for 5 minutes until it is browned. Place chicken in a clean bowl and set aside. DO NOT put the chicken back into the bowl it was in when it was raw.
3. Heat 1 tsp of olive oil at medium heat and add in the onion, garlic, chili and ginger. Cook it for ten minutes and turn on some ventilation—this will get spicy!
4. Add in the curry powder and 2 tsp of turmeric—Cook for another minute.
5. Mix in the canned tomatoes, coconut milk, cardamom pods, and ½ can of chicken stock. Reduce heat to barely above a simmer and wait 30 minutes
6. When the sauce is reduced, add the chicken and kale. Cook until kale has begun to wilt.
7. Serve over rice or buckwheat. Top it with a sprinkling of chopped cilantro.

Crispy Tofu Wraps

If you are needing a quick crunch but want lunch on the go, these wraps are perfect. They are healthy, and tofu is fantastic for you on a Sirtfood diet. Even better, you can add in kale and tomatoes for a sirtuin powerhouse lunch, all in the palm of your hand. This recipe involves baking your tofu rather than frying it so that it is healthier. All you have to remember to do is press the tofu before you bake it—meaning that you must make sure that you drain the liquid out so that it does not get soggy. Remove all of the liquid from the container and then set the tofu on paper towels and cover it, placing something on top of it, like a plate or a cutting board, with a heavy item right on top, leaving the cutting board to sit on top for 15 minutes to press out the liquid; otherwise, you risk getting soggy tofu!

Ingredients:

- 1 block of extra firm tofu (do not forget to drain and press it)
- 6 tbsp cornstarch
- 1/3 cup soy milk
- 1 cup of buckwheat, processed in a food processor until coarse and breadcrumb-like in texture
- 2 tbsp olive oil
- ½ tsp paprika
- 1 tsp oregano, dried
- Pinch of salt and pepper
- 6 whole wheat or whole grain wraps/tortillas
- Any toppings you want (tomatoes, kale, and arugula all work well)

To complete this recipe, you will do the following:

1. Turn your oven on and set it to 425 degrees Fahrenheit. Prepare a baking sheet with foil or parchment paper to prevent sticking.
2. Take your tofu and cut it up into roughly 24 bite-sized bits and set aside in a bowl.
3. Take another bowl, shallow this time, and combine your buckwheat crumbs, oil, and your seasonings. Mix until well combined.
4. Create an assembly line—you want to have tofu first, then cornstarch in a second shallow bowl, then your soy milk, and lastly, your buckwheat coating. Next to the coating, you should have your baking sheet ready.
5. Move along the assembly line with your tofu—dip first into cornstarch, coating it completely, then the milk, followed by the buckwheat crumbs. Make sure it is evenly coated and place on the baking sheet. Make sure that all tofu pieces are 2 inches apart to give them room—use a second sheet if you need to.
6. Bake for 25 minutes. Pull them out and turn all pieces over, then cook for another 10 minutes until firm and crispy.
7. Remove from oven and add to a wrap with toppings of your choice.

Kale Tofu Stir Fry

While stir fry is traditionally reserved for dinners a lot of the time, they can also keep quite well and create a wonderful meal that you can pack and take with you on the go every day at work; this means that if you really want to enjoy something tasty, full of veggies, and rich in antioxidants and sirtuins, this is the meal for you. This recipe is designed to serve four, meaning that you can use it all week if you want it for several meals, or you can cut the recipe in half if you want to do so.

Ingredients:

For the tofu:

- 1 block of firm tofu
- 3 tsp curry powder
- 2 tbsp soy sauce

For the stir fry:

- 3 large kale leaves, chopped
- 3 large arugula leaves, chopped
- ½ of a red cabbage
- 2 carrots, sliced
- 2 minced cloves of garlic
- 2 inches of minced ginger
- 4 tbsp soy sauce
- 4 servings of buckwheat noodles

To complete this recipe, you will need to do the following:

1. Start by cutting up your tofu. It should be in bite-sized pieces. Then, mix in the soy sauce and the curry powder for the tofu and create a paste, which you will use to coat the tofu cubes. Set aside.
2. Cook your buckwheat noodles according to the package. Set aside when they are done.
3. Prepare all of your vegetables.
4. Prepare two frying pans with oil and turn them up to high. Put the tofu in one pan and cook until golden on all sides.
5. Add your garlic and ginger to the other pan and saute for one minute
6. Add the kale, arugula, and cabbage to the garlic and ginger and cook until it begins to wilt. Then, add in the carrots and soy sauce. Cook for another two minutes.
7. Serve with pasta on the bottom, stir fry in the middle, and tofu on top, or store with pasta and stir fry in one container with the tofu in a separate one.

Salmon Salad

Want to add some salmon to your meal? This would be a great recipe to include with some, for example, wraps, or atop a bed of prepared buckwheat if you wanted to. It is a nice way to change things up and a simple lunch with canned salmon, tomatoes, and a sauce of olive oil and lemon juice. The simplicity of this meal is wonderful and enjoyable—just give it a try!

Ingredients:

- 12 ounces of canned salmon, drained
- ¼ cup diced tomatoes
- 4 green onions, sliced finely
- 2 tbsp olive oil
- 2 tbsp lemon juice
- A pinch of salt
- 1 can of chickpeas
- Pepper to taste

To complete this recipe, you will need to do the following:

1. Drain your tuna and chickpeas and add them to a bowl
2. Add in the tomato and green onions, then add the juice and salt and pepper. Combine well.
3. Serve over a bed of arugula and kale, in a wrap, or atop some buckwheat. It keeps for 2 days in the fridge.

Kale and Arugula Salad with Walnut Chicken

The kale and arugula combine with a nice, light dressing as well as some tasty, crispy chicken to create a sirtuin powerhouse that you can take with you to work with ease. This recipe is delicious, slightly spicy, and should keep you satisfied all day long.

Ingredients:

For the chicken:

- Olive oil to coat the pan
- 1 chicken breast
- 1 egg white
- 1/8 cup buckwheat flour
- ¼ cup ground walnuts
- 1 pinch of red pepper, ground
- ½ tsp dried parsley

For the salad:

- 1 cup arugula, chopped
- 2 cups kale, chopped
- ½ cup tomato, diced

Dressing:

- 1 tbsp lemon juice
- 1 green onion, minced
- 1 tsp honey
- 2 tbsp olive oil
- Salt and pepper to taste

To prepare this recipe, you will need to do the following:

- Prepare the chicken
    1. Preheat oven to 375 degrees Fahrenheit and coat a baking sheet with olive oil.
    2. Season your chicken breast with salt and pepper and set aside.
    3. In a bowl, add your egg white and beat it.
    4. In another bowl, add your buckwheat flour, your walnuts, your pepper, and your parsley.
    5. Take your chicken breast and dip it in the egg white. Then, coat it in the flour mixture until the whole chicken breast is covered. Place it on the baking sheet and spritz with olive oil.
    6. Bake for 20 minutes, or until internal temperature has reached 165 degrees Fahrenheit.

    7. Slice chicken and set aside.
- Prepare the dressing
    1. Mix your lemon juice, onion, and honey thoroughly. Then, slowly add in olive oil, mixing until combined.
- Prepare the salad
    1. In a salad bowl, combine your arugula, kale, and tomato. Mix until combined, then top with the dressing.
    2. Serve with a salad topped with sliced chicken.

Chapter 8: Dinner Recipes

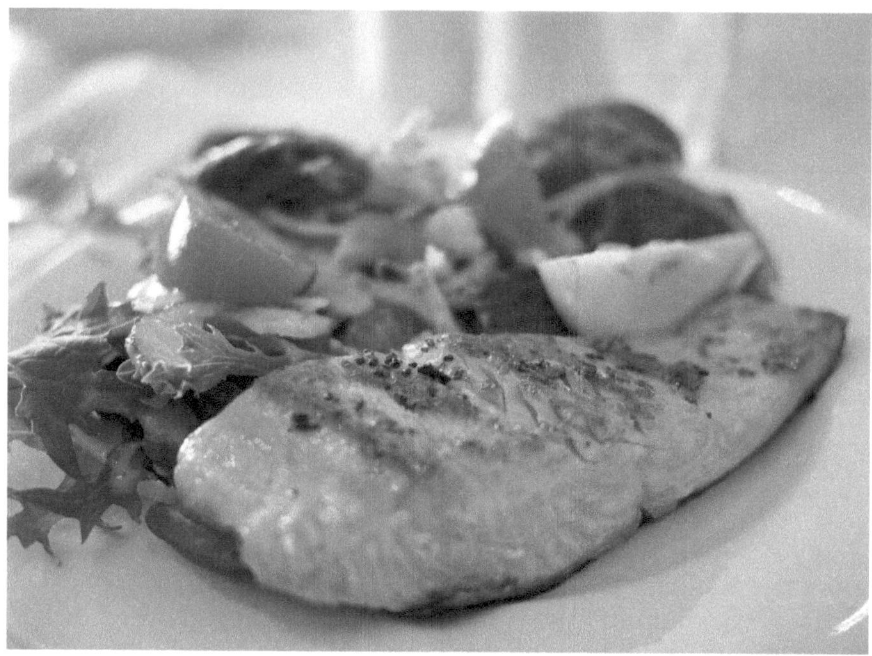

Dinner is one of the most important meals of the day—socially speaking. If you have a family, you probably all gather around the dinner table every evening to catch up on what everyone did that day, discussing what school was like, how work was, and more. Because of this, dinner recipes have to taste good—they should be pleasant to enjoy while you work through your day, and even better, you want to be able to share the recipes with your family as well. Now, let's take a look at ten recipes that you can enjoy, on your own or with family.

Turmeric Baked Salmon

Salmon is a delicious option for a protein that is full of all sorts of wonderful health benefits as well. From being full of omega-3 fatty acids that your body will thrive on to being coated with turmeric and lemon, and prepared with all sorts of other wonderful sirtfoods, this dish is here to make sure that you get a dish worth eating and enjoying.

Ingredients:

- 1 4 oz piece of salmon, skinned
- 1 tsp olive oil
- 1 tsp turmeric powder
- ¼ lemon, juiced

- ½ cup diced red onion
- 1/3 cup canned green lentils
- 1 clove of garlic, minced
- 1 bird's eye chili, minced (remove seeds if you do not like spicy foods)
- 1 ½ cups chopped celery
- 1 tsp curry powder (more to taste if you prefer it spicy
- ½ cup of chicken stock
- 1 tbsp chopped parsley
- 1 ½ small whole tomatoes, diced

To complete this recipe, you will need to do the following:

1. Preheat your oven to 400 degrees Fahrenheit.
2. Add olive oil to a frying pan on medium-low heat and wait until oil is shimmering. Then, add in onion, garlic, celery, ginger, and chili. Gently sauté for 2 or 3 minutes until it is softened. Then, add the curry powder and cook for another minute.
3. Add in the tomato, then the stock and finally, add in the lentils. Then, cook on low heat at a low simmer for 10 minutes. Check the texture of the celery to determine preference.
4. Mix turmeric, lemon juice, and oil together in a small bowl, then rub it on the salmon. Add it to a baking tray and cook for 10 minutes, or until flaking
5. Add parsley to the celery and serve with the salmon.

Prawn Stir Fry

Are you more of a prawn person? Thankfully, prawns are also a great option on the sirtfood diet and they are quite tasty. This meal will have you adding prawns to your buckwheat noodles and your veggies for a highly satisfying meal. This meal will serve a family of four and you may have to double it if the family likes the food—and it would be hard not to!

Ingredients

- 4 cups of raw shelled prawns, larger in size preferred, but any size will be fine
- 8 tbsp soy sauce
- 8 tbsp olive oil
- 10 oz of buckwheat noodles
- 4 cloves of garlic
- 4 bird's eye chili (less to taste or cut out the seeds to taste if you prefer it less spicy)
- 4 tsp fresh, minced ginger
- 2/3 cup of red onion, diced
- 1 1/3 cup celery, chopped
- 2 cups of green beans, chopped
- 3 cups of kale, chopped
- 2 cups of chicken stock

To complete this recipe, you will need to do the following:

1. Heat up a frying pan on high heat. Add the prawns with 4 tsp of soy sauce and 4 tsp of olive oil. Cook for 3 minutes and move prawns to a plate. Clean the pan with paper towels and set aside.
2. Prepare your noodles according to the packaging. Drain and set aside.
3. Add remaining oil to the frying pan and add in all of your vegetables. Cook at medium-high for 2-3 minutes and then add the stock.
4. Bring to a boil, then drop the temperature and allow it to simmer for two minutes. Then, add the prawns and the noodles. Bring back to a boil to warm them up and remove from heat.
5. Serve. This serves 4 people.

Chicken Zucchini Stir Fry

Sometimes, what we really need is something quick and easy, even when we are on a diet. After all, life waits for no one! When you need a quick meal, look no further—this dish will only take a few minutes and you will be able to enjoy it quickly. This dish will yield four servings in just 20 minutes of your time.

Ingredients:

- ¼ cup of soy sauce
- 1 cup of broth (chicken or veggie)
- 1 tbsp corn starch
- 2 tbsp mirin (Japanese sweet white wine)
- 1 tbsp honey
- 2 tsp sesame oil
- 1 tbsp olive oil
- 1 tbsp garlic, minced
- 1 tbsp ginger, minced
- 1 lb thinly sliced chicken breast
- 2 cups zucchini, sliced in thin half-circles
- Green onions for garnish

To complete this dish, you will need to do the following:

1. Add your soy sauce, broth, mirin, honey, sesame oil, and corn starch into a bowl and whisk thoroughly until well combined
2. Take a large frying pan or wok and add a teaspoon of olive oil on medium-high heat. Cook half of the chicken in one flat layer until cooked through—2-3 minutes per side. Then, set aside and repeat with the remaining half of chicken and another 1 tsp of oil.
3. Add in the last tsp of oil and the ginger and garlic. Cook until fragrant—roughly half of a minute. Then, stir in the sauce that you prepared in a bowl. Whisk well and cook for a minute. It should start to warm up and thicken.
4. Add zucchini and cook another two minutes until the zucchini is tender-crisp. Remove from heat and mix the prepared chicken into the mixture, coating well. Serve with green onions on top.

Prawn Arrabbiata

Once again, we are taking a look at a prawn dish—this one is deliciously enjoyable, spiced up with fragrant herbs that come together with a wine sauce to create a rich, enjoyable dinner for you. This recipe is quick and easy—and all you have to do is toss a few ingredients together.

Ingredients:

- 1 lb of shrimp, raw and shelled
- 10 oz buckwheat noodles
- 4 tbsp olive oil
- 1 ½ red onion, chopped finely
- 4 cloves of garlic, minced
- 1 cup of celery, diced
- 4 finely chopped bird's eye chili—remove seeds if you do not like it spicy
- 8 tbsp white wine
- 4 cups of canned crushed tomatoes
- 4 tbsp chopped parsley

To complete this recipe, you will need to do the following:

1. Start with sautéing the onions, chili, and celery in 4 tbsp of olive oil at medium-low heat for just a minute or two. Then, raise the temperature up to a medium and add the wine, cooking for another minute. Add in the tomatoes and leave it to simmer at medium-low for 30 minutes.
2. While the sauce simmers, prepare the pasta according to the packaging. Then, drain and toss with 1 tbsp of olive oil.
3. Add the prawns to the sauce and cook for four minutes, or until opaque. Then, add the parsley and pasta. Mix thoroughly and serve.

<u>Spiced Chicken Cauliflower Couscous</u>

If you want a quick and easy meal, this is another option, and even better, it is low carb thanks to the use of cauliflower for the couscous. This is delicious and the chili and the flavors will help even the most hesitant cauliflower haters enjoy this dish. This meal will feed two people and you can double it if you need to do so.

Ingredients:

- 1 ½ cups cauliflower, chopped in the food processor until roughly the size of rice
- 1 chicken breast
- 10 sprigs of parsley, chopped
- 2 tsp turmeric powder
- 1 clove of garlic, minced
- ¼ cup of carrots, diced
- ¼ cup red onions, finely diced
- 1 bird's eye chili, seeds removed and diced
- 1 tsp minced ginger
- 2 tbsp olive oil
- ¼ cup sun-dried tomatoes
- ½ lemon, juiced
- 1 tbsp capers

To prepare, you will need to do the following:

1. Prepare the cauliflower in a food processor and set it to the side
2. Add 1 tbsp of olive oil to a pan in medium-high heat and then add ginger, chili, onions, and garlic. Sauté until fragrant and soft.
3. Add the carrots and cauliflower, as well as the turmeric. Let it cook for 3 minutes.
4. Remove it from the heat and add it to a bowl that has the tomatoes and parsley. Set it to the side.
5. Use the remaining oil for cooking the chicken at medium heat until thoroughly cooked. Then, add lemon juice, water, and capers to the pan. Then, add the couscous and sauce in the same pan. Mix and serve with cilantro on top.

Instant Pot Chicken and Kale Curry

Here is yet another curry recipe for you featuring chicken and kale—but this one is for the instant pot. If you want to prepare your food in record time, this is a great option for you. Serve on rice or with buckwheat.

Ingredients:

- 3 tbsp olive oil
- 1 stick of cinnamon
- 2 cardamoms
- 2 cloves
- ¼ tsp fennel seed
- 4 tsp coriander powder
- 1 tsp cayenne powder
- ½ tsp turmeric
- 4 kale leaves, prepared and chopped
- 4 chicken thighs, boneless and skinned, chopped up to bites
- 2 cups of red onion, coarsely chopped
- 4 cloves of garlic, crushed then minced
- 1 tsp ginger, minced
- 1 cup of chopped tomato
- ½ cup canned light coconut milk
- 1 cup of water
- 2 tsp salt

To complete this recipe, do the following:

1. Turn your Instant Pot onto sauté, then add in the olive oil when it has heated up. Then, add in your whole spices (cinnamon, cardamom, clove, fennel). Let them cook for a few seconds until fragrant.
2. Then add in your onion, ginger, and garlic for 3-4 minutes, until your onions are beginning to become transparent.
3. Then, add in your tomato, coriander powder, and powdered spices. Allow it to sauté until the tomatoes have become soft and it is beginning to look like it is shimmering. Stir regularly, not allowing it to burn.
4. Turn off the instant pot and then stir in the chicken, kale, coconut milk, water, and salt. Set it to manual for 5 minutes and make sure that the valve is properly sealed.
5. After the 5 minutes, leave it in warm mode for another 4 minutes. Then vent and quickly release the pressure.
6. Taste and adjust flavor if necessary. Serve over buckwheat or rice.

Turmeric Chicken Kale Salad

Who said salads couldn't be a good option for dinner sometimes? If you want to have a nice, light meal for dinner, this is a great one for you, filled with all sorts of flavors and just as filling as it is nutritious.

Ingredients:

Chicken:

- 1 tbsp olive oil
- ½ onion, finely diced
- 9 oz of chicken, diced up
- 1 clove of garlic, minced
- 1 tsp turmeric
- 1 tsp lime zest
- ½ lime, juiced
- 1 tsp salt and pepper

Salad

- 2 cups of bite-sized broccoli florets
- 2 tbsp pumpkin seeds
- 3 leaves of kale, removing the stems and chopping them up
- ½ avocado, carefully sliced
- 1 handful of parsley and 1 handful of cilantro, roughly chopped

Dressing

- 3 tbsp lime juice
- 3 tbsp olive oil
- 1 minced clove of garlic
- 1 tsp honey
- ½ tsp Dijon mustard
- Salt and pepper to taste

To prepare, you will do the following:

1. Heat up the olive oil in a frying pan for the chicken on a medium to medium-high heat. Sautee the onion first at medium for a few minutes until the onions begin to turn golden—DO NOT LET THEM BURN. Burnt onion is bitter. Put the chicken in the pan and add the garlic. Stir it for 3 minutes on medium-high heat.
2. Then, add in the rest of your chicken ingredients and cook for 3-4 minutes, stirring regularly. Set it aside when it is done.

3. While waiting for the chicken to cook, boil a saucepan of water and cook the broccoli for just two minutes before shocking it in cold water and setting it aside.
4. Toast up your pumpkin seeds in the same pan you cooked your chicken for just two minutes on medium heat: season lightly and reserve for later.
5. Add your kale to a bowl, then add in the dressing. Use your hands to toss the kale, massaging in the dressing to help tenderize it.
6. Add the chicken, broccoli, pumpkin seeds, the fresh herbs, and avocado to the bowl and mix it through. Serve.

Lemon Garlic Salmon

One of the best parts of salmon is how quick and easy it is to cook—it is also wonderfully tasty, high in healthy fats and something that can be added to the menu with ease! If you like salmon, this recipe is for you. In particular, serve it atop some sautéed kale or arugula for additional sirtfood power.

Ingredients:

- 4 pieces of salmon, skin still attached
- A pinch of salt
- A pinch of pepper
- 2 tsp olive oil
- 1/3 cup of fresh-squeezed lemon juice
- 2 tbsp dill, fresh and finely topped
- 8 cloves of garlic, crushed and minced

This recipe is incredibly easy to throw together. All you have to do is the following:

1. Add a pinch of salt and pepper to the salmon
2. In a large skillet on medium-high heat, add olive oil and wait for it to shimmer. Then, place the salmon into the pan, skin side up. Wait three to four minutes, building a nice seared crust on the salmon and then flip it to sear the other side.
3. Push your salmon to one side of the pan and then add in the lemon juice and garlic. Let it sauté for a minute and then spoon it atop the salmon. Continue cooking until the fish flakes easily with the use of a fork.
4. Serve garnished with fresh dill atop the salmon.

Tofu and Mushroom Stir Fry

Are you looking for something vegetarian? This meal is for you. Whether you are vegetarian yourself or simply looking for a meatless meal, this is a great option that is tasty. It does help to press your tofu prior to beginning—leaving your tofu block between paper towels with something heavy to push down on the top to squeeze out extra water.

Ingredients:

- 1 block of tofu—extra firm and drained and pressed
- Rice or buckwheat for serving
- 1 lb. mushrooms of your choice
- 6 green onions
- 1 tbsp of ginger, minced
- 1 ½ tsp corn starch
- 2 tbsp rice vinegar
- ½ tsp red pepper flakes
- 2 tbsp mirin or white wine
- 3 tbsp soy sauce
- 2 tbsp olive oil

To complete this meal, you will need to do the following:

1. Prep all ingredients before beginning.
2. Add tofu, cut into small bite-sized pieces, into a bowl with the corn starch, pepper flakes, salt, and 1 tbsp soy sauce. Mix well.
3. In a small bowl, add the vinegar, wine, and last 2 tbsp of soy sauce and mix
4. Heat 1 tbsp of your oil into a skillet on medium-high and when it is ready, add in your mushrooms, green onions, and the ginger. Cook it while constantly tossing it for about 5 minutes, watching for the mushrooms to tenderize and brown. Sprinkle with salt and set aside in a bowl
5. Add 1 tbsp of oil in the skillet and heat. Add tofu in one layer without overlapping. Cook, without touching it for two minutes, then turn to the other side. Cook another two minutes.
6. Add your sauce and your mushrooms back into the frying pan and cook with regular stirring and tossing as the ingredients thicken about half a minute. Remove from heat and taste. Season as necessary. Serve.

Miso Sesame Glazed Tofu Stir Fry

And finally, one last tofu dish for another vegetarian option for dinner. This one could easily be made to be meat-based by substituting chicken for the tofu, but we are going to go over the recipe with tofu, specifically as a wonderful, soy-filled, sirtfood protein. This recipe will serve two in just about 40 minutes for a delicious dinner.

Ingredients:

- 2 tbsp white wine or mirin
- 2 tbsp brown miso paste
- 1 package of tofu
- 1 celery stalk, finely chopped and trimmed
- 1 red onion, in thin slices
- 1 zucchini, in thin half circles
- 2 bird's eye chili with seeds removed and diced. You can leave the seeds if you prefer spicier food
- 2 cloves of garlic, minced
- 1 ¼ cups kale, ribs removed and chopped
- 4 tsp sesame seed
- ½ cup buckwheat noodles
- 1 cup of water
- 2 tsp turmeric powder
- 2 tsp soy sauce
- 4 tsp olive oil

To complete this recipe, you will need to do the following:

1. Prepare a baking sheet with parchment paper and turn oven to 400 degrees F
2. In a bowl, add the wine and miso paste. Cut your piece of tofu horizontally, and then cut diagonally to create triangles. Marinate the tofu in the miso while you finish all prep work.
3. Prepare kale in a steamer for a few minutes, removing when wilting. Set aside.
4. Slice up your vegetables and set aside.
5. Put your tofu on your baking sheet and add the sesame seeds to the top. Bake for 20 minutes, looking for the nice caramelization to occur.
6. Prepare your buckwheat pasta according to the package instructions.
7. For the last 5 minutes of the tofu cooking, add olive oil to a frying pan and then sauté on high heat your vegetables for two minutes, then reduce to medium for another four minutes. The veggies should be cooked, but still, retain some bite to them. If the veggies begin to stick, add a bit of water.
8. Serve with veggies atop buckwheat pasta and tofu atop the veggies.

Chapter 9: Snack Recipes

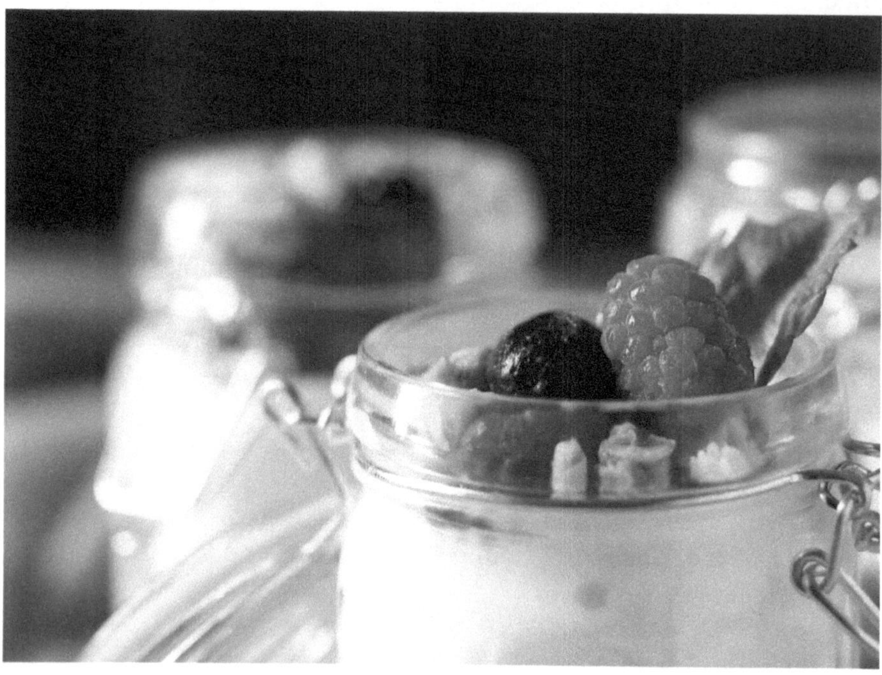

Even on a diet, we still get hungry sometimes. Maybe you are in maintenance mode and are not concerned with the hard and fast meal limit. That is perfectly fine if that is what works for you—and here are some snacks that you can use to be healthy and still rich in sirtfoods.

Creamy Turmeric Latte

Sometimes, all we need is a quick pick-me-up and this turmeric latte can do just that. It may not be caffeinated, but it sure packs an antioxidant punch to put a pep back in your step! This will create four lattes for you so that you can share them with all your friends!

Ingredients:

- 2 tsp turmeric powder
- 3/4 tsp cinnamon powder
- ½ tsp ginger powder
- ½ tsp vanilla powder (or vanilla extract in a pinch)
- 4 small pinches of black pepper for spice
- 4 ¼ cups of coconut milk, or any other alternative milk that you prefer

To complete this recipe, you will need to do the following:

1. Mix your herbs into a bowl with just a few tbsp. of milk to create a paste. Ix well, then divide among four mugs.
2. In a pan, heat your milk to just before boiling
3. Add the hot milk to the mugs and stir to integrate the paste.
4. Serve.

Kale Chips

Have you ever had kale chips? They are a great way to enjoy a bit of a crunch when you are missing potato chips but want something a bit healthier. This recipe will create a powerhouse of ingredients, all surrounding that kale to create a healthy, delicious, cheesy kale chip that you can enjoy, guilt-free.

Ingredients:

- 2 cup sunflower seeds
- 2 tbsp freshly squeezed lemon juice
- 1 teaspoon of turmeric powder
- 1/2 cup nutritional yeast
- Sea salt to taste
- ¼ cup of water if necessary
- 4 large kale bundles

To prepare this recipe, you must do the following:

1. The night before you are ready to create this recipe, put your sunflower seeds in a bowl and soak in water overnight.
2. When you are ready, drain the sunflower seeds. Add them to a food processor, along with the juice, yeast, and seasonings, as well as the water. Blend until it has a good consistency. Add more water if necessary to get a nice smooth consistency that can easily coat the kale.
3. Turn the oven on and set it to 225 degrees Fahrenheit, keeping in mind that convention baking will be useful here if you can.
4. On two baking sheets, set up some parchment paper.
5. Prepare the kale. Tear it into bite-sized, or chip-sized pieces, removing all of the large stems. Throw them all into a mixing bowl or two and coat the kale with the sunflower mix. Coat it as well as possible.
6. Put the kale on the baking sheets without overlapping or touching. This will often take several rounds through the oven to make it properly.
7. Bake for 20 minutes, turn the pans, toss the chips, and bake for another 20 minutes. They should become golden in color and crispy.
8. Remove and let cool.

Berry Parfait

What can be tastier than a berry parfait? These are wonderfully delicious, healthy, and refreshing. Try one of these parfaits for a quick snack if you need a short, sweet pick-me-up, or even try adding the next recipe, buckwheat granola, to it for something with a bit more density to it.

Ingredients:

- ½ cup of plain Greek yogurt
- ¼ cup diced strawberries
- ¼ cup diced blueberries
- Granola if desired
- Sweeten with a touch of honey if necessary

To complete this recipe, you will need to do the following:

1. Cut up your berries and set aside
2. Layer a small amount of berries in the bottom of a cup, followed by a small layer of yogurt. Repeat with berries and yogurt in several layers, adding honey if necessary or desired. Top with granola if desired.

Buckwheat Granola

For the times when you want a bit more crunch and something a bit more filling in the stomach, homemade buckwheat granola is a great option for you. Easy to make, easy to store, and easy to love, this makes a great power snack when needed.

Ingredients:

- 2 cups of uncooked buckwheat groats
- 1 ½ cup crushed walnut
- 4 tbsp sesame seeds
- Sprinkling of salt
- 2 tbsp olive oil
- 3 tbsp honey
- Dried Medjool dates

To complete this recipe, you will need to do the following:

1. Turn the oven to 325 degrees Fahrenheit and prepare a baking sheet with parchment paper to prevent sticking.
2. Atop the pan, add your buckwheat, walnuts, and sesame seeds. Gently sprinkle a touch of salt over everything and then add the oil and honey, mix thoroughly with your hands until well combined. Then, spread it out evenly.
3. Bake for 20 minutes, giving it a quick mix halfway through
4. Cool it on a counter and then add your dried dates. Store it in an airtight container.

Zucchini Tots

 Sometimes, we get a craving for something that we would eat before—like pizza, or in this case, tater tots. This recipe creates a healthy zucchini tot that you can enjoy guilt-free.

Ingredients:

- 1 cup of zucchini, shredded and packed
- 1 egg
- 1/3 cup of Italian cheese blend, shredded
- ¼ cup of Rice Chex, crushed up
- ¾ tsp Italian seasoning
- ¼ tsp garlic powder
- Salt and pepper to taste

To complete this recipe, you will need:

1. Turn the oven to 400 degrees Fahrenheit and allow to preheat
2. Measure out your zucchini and dry it out with a paper towel to remove moisture.
3. Combine bowl zucchini with all other ingredients and mix well.
4. Use a 2 tsp scoop to create tightly packed tots on parchment paper on a baking sheet. Bake for 25 minutes, turning halfway through.

Chapter 10: Treat and Dessert Recipes

Who says you can't have dessert when you're on a diet? This *is* the Sirtfood Diet, after all—one where chocolate is welcome! Let's go over five quick, delicious dessert recipes that you can make that are so deliciously decadent that you can hardly believe that you are eating healthily.

Healthy Brownie Bites

Healthy brownies—who knew you could get them? This particular brownie is made deliciously healthy with a mix of cacao powder, dates, and buckwheat flour. Give it a shot—you won't believe you're on a diet anymore after this!

Ingredients

- 14 large Medjool dates, pits removed
- 1 cup of hot water to soak the dated
- ¾ cup buckwheat flour
- ½ cup dark chocolate cacao powder
- ½ tsp baking powder
- 3 tbsp coconut sugar or honey
- 1 tbsp melted coconut oil
- 1 egg
- 2 tsp vanilla
- A sprinkling of salt
- Crushed walnuts for extra sirtuin power

To complete this recipe, you will need to do the following:

1. Turn the oven to 350 degrees Fahrenheit and while it is preheating, prepare an 8x8 or 9x9 baking pan with either nonstick spray or parchment paper
2. Soak your dates in hot water for 10 minutes. Blend the dates until they become smooth in consistency
3. Add your dried ingredients, coconut oil, vanilla, and the single egg to the blender. Blend it until it is well combined.
4. Add the batter to the pan and allow it to bake for 20 minutes until firm.
5. Top with walnuts if you want to do so.

Chocolate Coconut Bites

There is something incredibly satisfying about little bite-sized foods that are perfectly portioned. This particular one combines eight ingredients to create a delicious coconut ball that anyone can appreciate. This recipe will create a large yield and you and your family will not be able to get their fill!

Ingredients:

- 1 ½ cups of sliced almonds
- 1 cup of dark chocolate cocoa (unsweetened)
- 4 tbsp flax seeds (ground)
- Pinch of sea salt
- 2 2/3 cups of rolled oats
- 2 lbs of Medjool dates with the pits taken out
- ½ cup of melted coconut oil
- ½ cup of unsweetened, shredded coconut

To complete this recipe, you will do the following:

1. Add sliced almonds to the food processor and blend in a food processor to create a fine chop—20-30 seconds
2. To the food processor, add in your cocoa powder, your oats, your salt, and your flax seeds. Blend for 20 seconds.
3. Add in the dates and coconut oil and blend for 3 minutes, creating a well-blended batter. It should be thick and sticky enough to create balls.
4. Create 1 inch balls, shaping them in your hand. Place them on your baking sheet covered in parchment paper.
5. Add coconut shreds to a plate and press the balls into the coconut.
6. Enjoy—no baking required!

Chocolate Mousse

Now, let's take a look at a delicious chocolate soy mousse that even kids will go nuts for! Decadent and flavorful, these are healthy and full of those antioxidants and sirtuins.

Ingredients:

- 8 oz extra firm tofu, drained
- ¼ cup melted 85% dark chocolate
- 2 tbsp unsweetened dark chocolate cocoa powder
- ½ tsp vanilla
- ¼ cup honey or maple syrup
- ½ lemon, juiced
- ¼ cup of crystallized ginger (if you have it—optional)
- 1 cup of berries of choice for garnish

To complete this recipe, all you have to do is:

1. In a blender, add tofu, melted chocolate, cocoa powder, vanilla extract, syrup, and lemon juice. Blend until thoroughly incorporated and silky smooth.
2. Add in ginger, if desired.
3. Add to six small bowls or ramekins and top with the berries. Serve.

Chocolate Coffee Bites

Who doesn't love coffee and chocolate? This recipe brings them together—and even brings the nutritional powerhouse of unsweetened cocoa powder, dates, and coffee to you to create a delicious treat that will help to pack a sirtuin punch.

Ingredients:

- 4 Medjool dates pitted and prepared
- ¼ cup of espresso, cold
- ½ cup of almonds
- 2 tbsp dark chocolate cocoa powder
- ½ tbsp. chia seeds
- A tiny pinch of salt

To complete this recipe, you will do the following:

1. Soak your dates in coffee for 15-20 minutes. You want to drain the dates while still keeping the coffee for later.
2. Add dates to the food processor and pulse until smooth. Add 1 tbsp of the coffee to create a thick paste.
3. Add everything else to the processor and pulse until you create a dough.
4. Create small bite-sized balls and refrigerate them. Enjoy!

Conclusion

Congratulations! You have made it to the end of this book! Are you convinced yet? We have gone over dozens of healthy, delicious recipes that look like they would be enjoyable for just about anyone, and even better, they are packed with sirtuins! Remember, there is no commitment—you do not have to commit to the calorie restrictions if you do not want to, but the recipes in this book are healthy and delicious for anyone.

If you are ready to tackle the Sirtfood Diet and are preparing to move on to phase one, congratulations! You can do it! Remember that all diets are a bit difficult at first. It takes weeks to form a new habit, and while you may miss the old foods, you will learn to love and crave the new ones just as quickly. If you want to be able to enjoy your diet and really thrive, losing any weight that you have to kick off and learning to create the healthy lifestyle that you need, this is the book for you.

Stick to it! You can do it! You've already taken a monumental step just in picking up this book to read in the first place. Now, if you are ready, go look up a juicer. Start putting together your meal plans and shopping lists. Get ready to go on the journey of a lifetime, losing weight and feeling better than ever before!

Thank you so much for choosing this book to guide you through your journey to healthiness and wellness—hopefully, you feel like you have made the right one! If you have enjoyed this book, please consider heading over to Amazon to leave a review with your experience. It would be greatly appreciated! Good luck on your journey, and know that you have the power to make these great changes if you want it!